Belly Fat Breakthrough!

Smart Science for Transforming Your Body

KARLENE KARST, R.D.

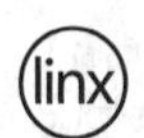

Printed in the United States of America

Books are available for special promotions and premiums.
For details, contact Special Markets, LINX, Corp., Box 613,
Great Falls, VA 22066, or e-mail specialmarkets@linxcorp.com.

ISBN-13: 978-1-9369610-0-9
ISBN-10: 1936961008
Book design by Paul Fitzgerald
Illustrations by Dee D'Amico
Copy editing by Ali Ferguson

Published by LINX

LINX, Corp.
Box 613
Great Falls, VA 22066
www.linxcorp.com

You should always consult with your doctor before making any changes to your diet or starting an exercise program.

contents

CHAPTER 1

Belly Fat Blues
What Causes It After All?

It just so happens that the first day I am working on this manuscript also happens to be January 3, 2011. I start my Monday morning after the holidays feeling a little sleepy and blah from all the holiday indulgences. So I start my day with a quick workout—well, what I think will be quick. As I walk into the gym, I hear the buzzing and humming of the cardio machines, the instructors motivating and belting out to their clients who are sweating away in their zumba, spinning, and step classes. My heart immediately quickens, and I feel that rush of excitement of being surrounded by like-minded in-shape individuals. Wow, if only the gym was like this every day. This signals the start of the new year, and everyone's new year's resolution is apparently to exercise in an attempt to lose weight once and for all. I smile to myself because I know by the end of the month, the gym will still be busy, but it will pretty much be the regulars, and I get it. It isn't fun. Exercising is hard work. It seems like only if you are in shape, can exercising be remotely fun. I love the sweat, the feeling of euphoria that follows my workout. But this is probably because outside of a few pregnancy pounds left to lose, I haven't had a weight problem. Why is this? Is it genetics? Is it good luck or more importantly good management? I believe it's the latter. I am lucky to have a personal interest in health and nutrition, so as a result, I have spent my post-secondary education and life living and eating healthfully. In fact, it is really just second nature, and I don't give it too much thought. For me, exercise has always been a part of my life, and I really like it; it is my stress release, my alone time, and a way to connect with my body for just a few hours a week. I used to be able to log more cardio hours, but since becoming mommy, I am happy to fit it in whenever I can. Instead, exercise now involves my two boys—packing them up into the stroller or putting them in the baby carrier. I really want to instill in them how important it is to get fresh air and to keep healthy and exercise.

However, I am not here to tell you that losing weight is easy because I know it's not. What I am hear to do is remind you of a growing and dangerous problem—belly fat—and give you some important food, exercise, and supplement tips that when combined, will prove to be the winning combination for beating belly fat once and for all.

OUR GROWING WAIST LINES

Why would you want to buy and read another book on belly fat? The fact remains that we have ominous statistics everywhere we turn:

- The rates of obesity are climbing, and the percentage of children and adolescents who are obese has doubled in the last 20 years.
- Some researchers have estimated that obesity causes about 300,000 deaths in the United States annually.
- Obesity is fueling an epidemic of type 2 diabetes, which also reduces individuals' lifespan.
- The prevalence of obesity in U.S. adults has increased about 50% per decade since 1980.
- According to a *New England Journal of Medicine* report, studies suggest that two-thirds of American adults are overweight (having a body mass index (BMI) of 25 or more) or obese (having a BMI of 30 or more).
- 30% of adults age 20 and over are obese.
- 15% of children age 6-11 and 30% age 12-19 are obese.
- Obesity costs $117 billion a year.

APPLE GONE BAD? TRY A PEAR!

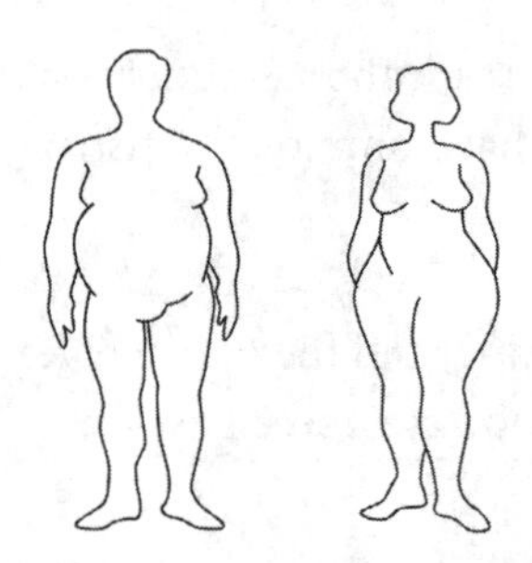

There is considerable variability in the relationship between obesity and chronic disease. Individuals with an "apple," or abdominal, fat distribution are at a substantially higher risk of developing cardiovascular problems compared with those with a "pear," or lower body, fat distribution pattern. Big hips are better than a big stomach, especially when it comes to heart disease, insulin resistance, and diabetes. Although genetics plays a major role in determining body shape, gender and age are also important factors. Men are typically the ones to end up with the spare tire, or belly fat, and women are usually the ones to gain excessive weight around the buttocks. After menopause, as estrogen supplies dwindle, women start storing fat around their abdomen, becoming more apple-shaped in the process and increasing their risk of cardiovascular disease and type 2 diabetes.

WAIST TO HIP RATIO—NOT THE SCALE

You can breathe a sigh of relief now; you are not going to be required to weigh yourself if you don't want to. In fact, I rarely know my weight, outside of my two pregnancies.

It really is unimportant. You know if you are carrying an excess of fat without even stepping on the scale. You can tell when you look in the mirror and of course by the way your clothes fit. Once you start this program start losing fat (not just weight), and begin increasing your lean muscle, you will find that you will shrink in size, but your overall weight on the scale might not even change. This is because muscle weighs more than fat, but muscle cells take up less space than fat cells, so you will find your body shrinking. What is important is not how much weight you carry, per se, but where you carry your weight. Research on obesity and its co-diseases, such as cardiovascular disease and type 2 diabetes, shows us that belly fat is the most dangerous of all. Carrying weight in the upper half of your body (like an apple) is far more dangerous than having a big bum (like a pear).

One way to know if you're an apple or a pear is to measure your waist-to-hip ratio by dividing your waist measurement (at the narrowest point) by your hip measurement (at the widest point). Women with waist-to-hip ratios of more than 0.8 and men with waist-to-hip ratios of more than 1.0 are apples and are at increased health risks due to their fat distribution. An even simpler method is to remember the ideal waist size (measured at your belly button) for a woman is 32.5 inches, and over 37 inches increases your risk of disease. For men, 35 inches is the ideal waist size, and anything over 40 will put you at a greater risk of heart disease, type 2 diabetes, and other weight-related problems.

All people who are obese are, to some degree, insulin resistant. However, people with belly fat are far more insulin resistant. Why? One hypothesis is that the fat tissue from the belly is more metabolically relevant.

FAT CELLS ARE THE KEY

The human body contains approximately 30 billion fat cells. Basically we all have the same amount of fat cells, but the difference between individuals is how much fat is stored in each of their fat cell. Our fat cells have an unlimited ability to keep expanding; they just grow and grow and grow. So how can we stop our fat cells from expanding?

First of all, we need to discuss the different types of fat in the body. There seem to be so many fat words floating around—white fat, brown fat, omentum fat, subcutaneous fat, and visceral fat—and the list keeps going on. Because belly fat loss is the key argument here, we will focus on the types of fat that are found in this region.

Subcutaneous Fat

Subcutaneous fat, or white fat, is the insulating layer of fat just beneath the skin that buffers us from the cold and stores calories. Despite the fact that women have more total body fat than men, because females' fat is primarily subcutaneous, they don't have the rates of metabolic syndrome and heart disease that men do. An important message is that belly fat and insulin resistance have a dual relationship. Belly fat stimulates insulin resistance, and insulin resistance promotes belly fat.

Omentum Fat

Dr. Oz made the term omentum fat famous during an episode of Oprah on which he showed a healthy and fatty omentum. Neither was a pretty sight. The greater omentum sits in front of the stomach, while the lesser omentum covers the liver. Both easily store fat. Have you ever wondered why some men look almost, dare I say, pregnant? It's because the omentum in the front of the stomach may make the abdomen appear stiff and distended when it is large, resembling a pregnant belly. Men have higher levels of intra-abdominal fat than women do—in fact women have one-half the level. Thus, in men, this expanded omentum can get so hard and large that it resembles a woman in her seventh month of pregnancy. The goal is to lose this dangerous belly (omentum) fat, and when it shrinks, it reduces the risk of many diseases. One of the other dangers of a fatty omentum that covers the liver is that it can start the inflammatory process, which leads to cardiovascular disease, type 2 diabetes, and certain types of cancer. The fat that is released from the omentum travels to your liver (remember it sits on top of it) where it can cause an increase in lousy cholesterol (LDL), which is why the fat on your bum and thighs matters little in comparison to your belly fat. Remember an apple shape is more dangerous to your health than a pear shape.

CAUSES OF BELLY FAT

Excess Calories

Data from the United States and Canada show that overall food consumption is increasing, including increased soft-drink consumption and increased sugar consumption overall.

In particular, people are eating out more. This increase in eating food away from home, particularly in fast-food restaurants, is not surprising considering that in the United States, the number of fast-food restaurants grew 147% from 1972 to 1995 and the percentage of meals and snacks consumed at fast-food restaurants doubled. Eating at fast-food restaurants is associated with increased calorie and fat intake—largely due to increases in high-fat, high-sugar food choices, such as French fries and soft drinks, and decreases in consumption of fruits, vegetables, and milk. Aside from fast-food restaurants, even our grocery store environments have changed. The shift from small grocery stores in neighborhoods to large supermarkets has been positively associated with increased caloric intake because these supercenters offer a greater variety of processed and convenience foods.

An increase in our calories can also be partly blamed on growing portion sizes. Examinations of trends in food portion sizes in the United States from 1977 to 1998 revealed that portion sizes and energy intake increased for all key foods (except pizza) in all locations with the largest portions consumed at fast-food restaurants. The "super sizing" of portions is one of the greatest contributors. For example, the current McDonald's "child size" soft drink is 12 ounces; the same serving size in the 1950s would have been marketed as "king size." A recent study showed that the serving sizes recommended by the USDA and those currently being sold in restaurants shows have increased in size and now exceed the standards: soda by 35%; fast-food hamburger by 112%; bagel by 195%; steak by 224%; and cookie by 700%. Portion sizes began to grow in the 1970s, although fewer than 10 large-sized portions were introduced in that decade. The number of larger sizes rose sharply in the 1980s and has continued to increase steadily. Between 1995 and 1999, 65 new large-size portions were introduced.

However, as we all know, there are many other causes of being overweight than simply eating a few too many sweets and too many calories. While the causes of obesity are not totally understood, it is a known fact that there are endless factors leading to this problem, some which appear to be very simple and others very complicated.

The following causes, however, seem to be the most important factors of obesity:

- Genetics
- Sedentary lifestyle
- Lack of Sleep
- Stress
- Hormones (excess estrogen)
- Blood sugar imbalances (insulin resistance)
- Healthy fat deficiencies
- Poor diet
- Sympathetic nervous system
- Environmental toxins

Genetics

Complex interactions between genes and our environment exist. Obesity would not be possible if the human genome did not have the genes for it. Genes make obesity possible, but eating too many calories over time is also necessary to realize that potential. Genetic contributions are estimated to contribute 20-75% of variability in body weight.

The "thrifty gene hypothesis" suggests that people developed strong biological mechanisms for conserving energy as fat to enable their survival in times of famine. In times of plenty, such as the present day, the thrifty gene promotes obesity. The complex gene-environment interaction is clearly implicated in the obesity epidemic, as the rapid increase in obesity suggests an environment that promotes obesity more so than in the past. According to the World Health Organization (WHO), however, the fundamental causes of the obesity epidemic are societal, resulting from an environment that promotes an inactive lifestyle and the consumption of too many calories.

Sedentary Lifestyle

Sedentary lifestyle is one of the principal causes for excess belly fat and overall obesity. Further, it has been proven that physical activity is one of the greatest ways to use body energy.

Increased physical activity allows enables us to intake more calories and achieves a more favorable caloric balance in the body to avoid excess belly fat. Data from the National Nutrition Health and Examination Survey III (NHANES III) reports that 25% of the population partakes in no physical activity, while another 44% report not partaking in regular physical activity. A Nurse's Health Study conducted in the United States from 1992 to 1998 documented new cases of obesity and diabetes among subjects and correlated the outcomes with the participants' sedentary behaviors. Each two-hour/day increment in TV watching was associated with a 23% increase in obesity and a 14% increase in diabetes risk. The authors of the study also noted that each one-hour/day of brisk walking was associated with a 24% reduction in obesity and a 34% reduction in diabetes. This supports the premise that decreasing sedentary behaviors and increasing active leisure time reduces individuals' risk of obesity.

We will discuss physical activity in greater detail in Chapter 7.

Sleep

Sleep deprivation is increasingly being linked to the obesity epidemic. Research shows that obese people sleep less than their normal-weight peers. Insufficient sleep has been associated with changes in hormone levels that may stimulate appetite. In a study published in *Archives of Internal Medicine* in 2005, researchers found that people with a normal BMI slept 16 minutes more per day than obese people. Thus, even an extra 20 minutes of shuteye can be beneficial. Those who slept less were also found to have 15% less leptin—a hormone that suppresses appetite (this will be discussed in more detail in the next chapter).

Stress

The role of stress and belly fat is a well-documented problem. The hormone cortisol is secreted by the adrenal glands in response to physical, psychological, or environmental stress. If you experience chronic stress, your cortisol levels will remain elevated. The omentum also receives and stores hormones like cortisol, and high stress can stimulate the growth of the omentum. In fact, people who are under a lot of stress may find it very difficult to shrink the size of their omentum. For these individuals, losing belly fat is not going to be about just changing food habits; they will also have to restructure their lifestyle to include more relaxation and stress-reducing exercises. In addition, research now correlates chronically elevated cortisol levels with blood sugar problems, fat accumulation, fatigue, heart disease, and making fat cells resistant to fat loss. Further, if you have high cortisol levels, you will also likely require adrenal support as a result of the excess stress making cortisol places on the adrenal glands.

Hormone Balancing

Hormones have a powerful influence on weight gain and belly fat, and the hormone products from fat cells play a role in the insulin resistance of obese individuals. In particular, leptin is a hormone secreted by fat cells that is thought to cause satiety, the feeling of having eaten enough, and to stimulate the metabolic rate. Another hormone, ghrelin, is a powerful appetite-stimulating hormone and has been found in very high concentrations in the central nervous systems of obese individuals. Adiponectin is an important hormone that stimulates insulin sensitivity and has anti-inflammatory effects—two of the central factors required to prevent excess belly fat. Obese people secrete less adiponectin than do non-obese people. Working in just the opposite fashion is resistan, which decreases insulin sensitivity. The ideal scenario is to have high levels of adiponectin and leptin and low levels of ghrelin and resistan.

Free fatty acids are the primary breakdown of fat cell nutrient stores. Obesity increases levels of free fatty acids; thus, the overall release of free fatty acids into the blood stream is also a function of fat mass. An obese person will have higher total free fatty acid release than a thin person even if each fat cell releases the same quantity of free fatty acids. This may contribute to higher circulating free fatty acid levels and insulin resistance in obese individuals. The adverse effects of high free fatty acids extend beyond insulin resistance, which will be discussed in more detail in the next chapter.

So overall, when it comes right down to it, there are many causes, reasons, and even excuses for why so many people are carrying excess belly fat. The intention of the remainder of this book is to help you overcome any excuses in order to make losing belly fat a part of your everyday life and part of a lifestyle change. Remember, for whatever program you start on—be it the latest fad diet, Weight Watchers, Jenny Craig, or just good old nutrition advice—please be sure you think it is something you can continue doing for at least a year. If you think the plan you are on will last a month, then it isn't the right plan for you. To be successful, this must be a lifestyle change. It isn't an option anymore; it's a must. Belly fat is real, and belly fat is dangerous, but the good news is that we can banish belly fat. Are you ready?

CHAPTER 2

Hunger Hormones

In 2010, *Women's World* printed 10 cover issues with the headline "the dangers of belly fat," over 50 books were written on this topic last year alone, and everyone from Dr. Oz to Travis Stork of the hit show "The Doctors" is trying to educate us on the dangers of belly fat. Finally, it seems like we have found a word and topic that everyone can relate to. Why? Because it seems that no matter where we are or who we look at, most of us are harboring far too much weight in our midsection.

INSULIN—THE KEY HORMONE FOR BELLY FAT GAIN AND LOSS

After you consume carbohydrates, your blood sugar levels rise. As the regulator of blood sugar levels, insulin's job is to push glucose into the cells. On the surface of the cells are insulin receptors, which act like little doors that open and close to regulate the inflow of blood sugar.

When the body is continually blasted by foods containing high levels of simple sugars, the cells are bombarded with so much insulin that these doors begin to malfunction and shut down. With fewer doors open, the body needs to produce even more insulin to push glucose into the cells because insulin left free in the bloodstream cannot perform its function of lowering sugar levels. As a result of sugar's continued presence, the pancreas is stimulated to produce more insulin, and a vicious cycle is in place, resulting in a condition called insulin resistance.

With insulin resistance, the blood insulin levels are chronically high, which inhibits our fat cells from giving up their energy stores to let us lose weight. The more overweight we are, the more resistant to insulin we tend to become. This happens because extra fat causes a hormone reaction that closes the cells' doors to incoming glucose. High insulin leads to more fat cells (which are inefficient glucose burners) and fewer lean muscle cells. More fat cells means more belly fat, less ability or desire to exercise, and therefore less glucose burned. This is why some people gain more weight than others. However, the good news is that as we lose body fat, especially around the belly, our insulin resistance improves.

Insulin Stores Fat

To understand why insulin is such a critical component of belly fat, it is important to understand the relationship between food, blood sugar, insulin, and fat.

The human body is designed to do one of three things with the food we consume: 1) burn some of the calories as immediate energy, 2) store what is not utilized immediately in its 30 billion fat cells, or 3) store some of the excess sugars as short-term energy—referred to as glycogen (long chains of sugar molecules)—within the liver and skeletal muscles.

Herein lies the problem. The average human body only requires about one level teaspoon (5 grams) of blood sugar at any one time to run its millions of biochemical reactions. At the same time, our bodies have the ability to store only about half a day's worth of glycogen, which means that we have a very limited storage capacity for sugar.

By over-consuming the wrong types of carbohydrates (not those found in fruits and vegetables, which also contain fiber), you generate a rapid increase in blood sugar levels, in turn causing the pancreas to pump out loads of insulin. Insulin is essentially a storage hormone that not only lowers blood sugar but also sends a powerful message to your fat cells—STORE FAT!

Insulin accomplishes this task by stimulating a very powerful fat-storing enzyme called lipoprotein lipase (LPL), which expands fat cells while simultaneously making sure that fat doesn't get used as a fuel source. LPL is so good at its job, in fact, that many obesity researchers refer to it as the gatekeeper of fat storage.

Since our bodies have only a limited capacity to store carbohydrates, any carbohydrates not used immediately by the body or stored as glycogen are converted into triglycerides and are stored within our 30 billion fat cells throughout the body with the aid of LPL (and insulin). So, as you can see, a food does not have to contain fat to become fat in the body.

Just as we set the tone for continual fat storage through poor dietary choices (excessive amounts of high-glycemic carbohydrates), inactivity, insufficient sleep, and excess stress, we can also create the proper environment for continual fat loss by moving our bodies more; reducing stress; sleeping approximately eight hours each night; avoiding fat-storing (processed) carbs; and consuming more fruits, vegetables, high-quality proteins—including grass-fed varieties of beef, game meat, organic free-run chicken, organic eggs, fish—and good fats (safflower oil, fish, flax, hemp, almonds, and walnuts).

Insulin Triggers Fat Storage

Our bodies are not designed to handle an abundance of high-glycemic carbohydrates. After our bodies reach their capacity to use carbohydrates, they convert them into fat, which, coupled with our sedentary lifestyle, is a recipe for belly fat. This refined carbohydrate overload leads to the development of insulin resistance.

Do You Have Insulin Resistance?

The diagnosis of insulin resistance is fairly simple. Place a check by any item that applies to you:

- Do you have family history of diabetes, being overweight, abnormal cholesterol or triglycerides, high blood pressure, or heart disease?

- Do you crave sugary or starchy foods frequently?
- Is it difficult for you to lose weight, especially around your middle?
- Do you feel that you are addicted to carbohydrates?
- Do you experience shakiness, difficulty thinking, or headaches (often in the afternoon) that go away after you eat?
- Do you have afternoon fatigue?
- Have you experienced hypoglycemia?
- Is your Body Mass Index (BMI) greater than 30? (see Chapter 9.)
- Are you ten pounds or more over what you would call your "ideal" weight?
- Do you exercise fewer than two times per week?
- Are you of Native American, Asian, African-American, or Hispanic ancestry?
- Do you have high blood pressure?
- Do you have high triglycerides and low HDL cholesterol?
- Are you 45 years old or older?
- Have you had a history of gestational diabetes in pregnancy?
- Do you have polycystic ovary syndrome?

- Have you ever experienced acanthosis skin changes—velvety, mossy, flat, wart-like darkened skin on your neck or armpits or underneath your breasts?
- Do you smoke?

If you answered yes to three or more of these questions, you are likely insulin resistant. The more yes answers you gave, the more likely you are to have insulin resistance and the greater your risk is of developing health problems, such as type 2 diabetes and cardiovascular disease.

What can be done to control insulin resistance?

- Limit your intake of simple carbohydrates and choose low-glycemic carbohydrates *(see Chapter 4)*.
- Combine carbohydrates with a protein at every meal and snack.
- Eat five to six small meals per day.
- Replace one or two meals per day with a protein shake.
- Exercise regularly and include cardiovascular exercise and weight training. Controlling body fat is more important than losing

pounds. Remember that muscle is more metabolically active than fat. Even when you are sitting around doing nothing, muscle burns more calories than fat, so any increase in lean muscle will make your body a more efficient fat-burning machine.

- Use nutritional supplements (see Chapter 8).
- Incorporate high linoleic acid safflower oil (SafSlim™) into your supplement regime.

These actions are not optional or negotiable. Your body will burn fat (and properly utilize nutrients) only if your metabolism is balanced.

BAD BELLY FAT HORMONES TRIGGER BELLY FAT ACCUMULATION

Now that you understand why it's so important to keep insulin levels balanced, we can talk about some of the other important hormones that are involved in increased belly fat.

Insulin is the promoter of fat storage and shuttles fat to the belly region. Resistin is another important hormone that resists the action of insulin and is released from belly fat. The more fat you have, the more resistin will be released, which reduces cells' sensitivity to insulin and causes the insulin receptor sites (doors on the cells) to stay closed. As a result, sugar from our food will stay in the bloodstream, causing an even greater spike of insulin to try and push it back into the cells. The more circulating insulin, the more fat will be stored. It really is a vicious cycle.

Good Belly Fat Hormones Activate Belly Fat

Thankfully, there are hormones that can help our waist line, not just hinder it. Released from fat cells, adiponectin is a hormone that improves insulin sensitivity and can help mobilize belly fat. Thus, the goal is to have high levels of adiponectin. The less fat you have, the more adiponectin is released. If you have a lot of belly fat, only a small amount of adiponectin will be released, which causes our cells to become resistant to insulin and will, in turn, cause more fat to be stored in the belly region. Adiponectin also has anti-inflammatory effects on the cells lining the walls of the blood vessels. As a result, high blood levels of adiponectin are associated with a reduced risk of heart attack. Unsurprising, low levels of adiponectin are found in people who are obese (and who are at an increased risk of a heart attack).

Hunger Hormones

At 5:00 p.m. when your stomach is growling, the hormone ghrelin is calling you to feed your body. Ghrelin is a hormone found in the stomach lining and was actually discovered in obese individuals during gastric bypass surgery. It is responsible for stimulating the appetite and has been found to increase the appetite before eating and to decrease it afterward. Ghrelin also slows the metabolism and decreases the body's ability to burn fat. It doesn't matter how hard you try to ignore the calling of hunger, the hormone ghrelin is going to win every time. This is why it's important to continually fuel your body, so that an excessive amount of ghrelin is not released. If you keep your blood sugar balanced, ghrelin will stay under control and will not cause your metabolism to slow down in order to conserve energy. The last thing our belly fat needs is for the body to slow down the use of fat for energy.

The opposite of ghrelin is leptin, which is produced in fat cells and helps reduce appetite and increase our body's metabolism. There are numerous things we can do to help improve leptin levels:

- Eat five to six small meals per day. This enables your blood sugar to remain balanced, which helps the body secrete more leptin.
- Eat high-quality protein with carbohydrate foods. Protein foods are partly responsible for the feeling of satiety.
- Incorporate a high linoleic acid safflower oil like SafSlim™, which research has shown to decrease belly fat and improve the levels hormones associated with burning belly fat.

In the next chapter, we will look at how food impacts the belly fat hormones and causes increased weight gain.

CHAPTER 3

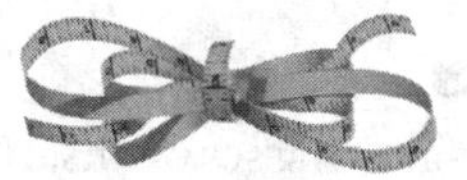

The Skinny on Fat

Major changes in the type and amount of fats we consume have occurred over the past 40-50 years. Diets high in the wrong types of fat make belly fat and insulin resistance worse by interfering with the burning of glucose and increasing insulin resistance. So what kinds of fats should we be consuming?

There are some fats that are necessary for the body to function, and you should include them in your diet. These are unsaturated fats—namely, the essential fatty acids. Then, there are the bad fats that most of us eat every day, which increase our risk of heart disease, diabetes, belly fat, and inflammation. Thus, in order to reach your weight goals, it is important to understand which fats should be included in your meals in order to prevent belly fat and insulin resistance.

GOOD FATS: ESSENTIAL FATTY ACIDS

Unsaturated Fats

There are three major classes of unsaturated fats: omega-3, omega-6, and omega-9. The omega-3s and omega-6s are polyunsaturated, and they are an essential part of our diet because the body cannot make them. Polyunsaturated fats include borage, evening primrose, corn, flaxseed, safflower, sunflower, sesame, fish oil, fatty fish, nuts, and seeds.

The omega-9s (found in olive oil), also known as oleic acid, are monounsaturated and nonessential (because the body can make them from other fats), yet, they are still a very healthy type of fat, and one that you should emphasize in your diet. In fact, olive oil has been found to help decrease insulin resistance and achieve healthier cholesterol levels.

Functions of Essential Fatty Acids

The three main functions of essential fatty acids (EFAs) are to regulate cellular processes, influence membrane function and integrity, and produce hormones that regulate and balance inflammation.

Cell Membrane Integrity

EFAs are integral components of cell membranes, determining fluidity and other physical properties as well as affecting structural functions—for example, the maintenance of enzyme activity. Our bodies are built of billions of cells, which, in turn, are built of membranes, and membranes are built of fats. Cell membranes built with polyunsaturated essential fats are less rigid and more fluid than membranes built with saturated fats. Fluid cells are extremely important for many reasons: they enable the transport of valuable nutrients into cells; they help keep toxins out of cells; they elasticize tissue; they expand blood vessel walls to reduce heart workload; they improve the overall function of organs; they influence sensitivity; they help your body utilize the insulin made by your pancreas; and they help control glucose levels.

If your cells are built of saturated fats, they will become rigid and hard. You may not notice the effects of your diet and its role in your health when you are young, but if you continue to consume a diet full of unhealthy fats, you will start to see the effects manifested in inflammatory conditions like arthritis, insulin resistance, metabolic syndrome, cardiovascular disease, and diabetes. It is extremely important that your cells are built of healthy fats, which keep the cells fluid.

The Power of Hormones

Some of the most potent effects of EFAs are related to their conversion into a series of eicosanoids, or hormones. These hormones function as intracellular communication agents that control the balance of virtually every system in the body, including the mechanisms for inflammation, blood clotting, and blood vessel dilation.

Bad Omega-6s and Excess Belly Fat

Many people with excess belly fat have a dietary condition in which the eicosanoid (hormone) pathways begin producing pro-inflammatory hormones. This may result from dietary a deficiency of certain polyunsaturated fats or from alterations in the ratio of omega-6s and omega-3s. Studies show that EFAs can affect the release of insulin. The insulin-releasing effect of fats decreases with the degree of unsaturation, meaning that the more saturated a fat is, the less chance the pancreas has of releasing insulin, which is why polyunsaturated fats do a better job of enabling insulin secretion.

Numerous theories have been suggested to explain the relationship between fats and insulin resistance, including changes in membrane fluidity, the number of insulin receptor sites, and increased activity in insulin receptors (polyunsaturated fats make insulin receptor sites more active). Research has shown that as the omega-6/omega-3 ratio decreases, insulin resistance improves.

Omega-6 Linoleic Acid and Belly Fat Loss

Exciting new research done at the University of Ohio in 2009 shows how safflower oil that is high in linoleic acid (different than the commercially available grocery store variety, which is high in oleic acid and is suitable for cooking) was beneficial in reducing belly fat. The researchers compared two oils: one had conjugated linoleic acid, which previous research has proven reduces BMI and overall body fat, and the other was high linoleic acid safflower oil. As studies have continually proven that belly fat is the most dangerous type of fat, researchers wanted to determine if changing the type of oil used would help target the dangerous intra-abdominal fat.

The results of this study were impressive. Safflower oil was found to reduce fat in the belly (trunk) area by 6.3% (2-4 pounds of belly fat), lowered blood sugar, and increased lean muscle.

All of the women in the study took one of the oils for 16 weeks followed by the other oil for an equal amount of time. The women did not change their diets or exercise routines, so researchers were able to measure the effects of only supplementation.

Another amazing result of the study was how safflower oil increased the hormone adiponectin. Researchers believe that an increase in this hormone may improve the body's ability to burn dietary fats, and adiponectin increases insulin sensitivity. Body fat decreases this extremely important hormone, and generally speaking, the more fat a person has on their frame, the lower his/her levels of adiponectin. However, consuming high linoleic acid safflower oil helps the body improve levels of adiponectin, which, in turn, causes the body to reduce body fat. The less body fat, the more adiponectin.

A new product called SafSlim™, which utilizes an emulsified high linoleic acid safflower oil, has recently been launched (see Chapter 8 for more information).

This is a delicious and convenient way for individuals to increase healthy linoleic acid and reduce body fat.

Omega-3 and Belly Fat Loss

Other research has found omega-3s to be powerful weight-loss agents. These researchers confirmed many ways in which omega-3s help with weight loss:

- Fish oil omega-3s stimulate the secretion of leptin, a hormone that decreases appetite and promotes fat burning.
- Fish oil omega-3s enable the burning of dietary fats by helping the body move fatty acids into body cells for burning as fuel.
- Fish oil omega-3s encourage the body to store dietary carbohydrates in the form of glycogen rather than as hard-to-lose body fat.
- Fish oil omega-3s reduce inflammation, which is known to promote weight gain.
- Fish oil omega-3s enhance blood sugar control by increasing insulin-producing cells' sensitivity to sugar.
- Fish oil omega-3s flip off genetic switches that promote inflammation and the storage of food as body fat.
- Fish oil omega-3s help the body transport glucose from the blood to cells by increasing the fluidity of cell membranes.

Good Foods with Good Fats

Healthy fats are easily consumed from a variety of delicious sources. Avocadoes, dark green leafy vegetables, fatty fish, nuts, seeds, olives, and unrefined expeller-pressed oils are rich in EFAs and can protect you from obesity, insulin resistance, metabolic syndromes, and the consequences of these problems—diabetes and heart disease.

Ways to Increase Good Fats in Your Diet

- Eat cold-water fatty fish, such as wild salmon, tuna, mackerel, sardines, or anchovies two times per week. The American Heart Association recommends this to prevent heart disease. If you don't like the taste of fish, try a toxin-free fish oil supplement.
- Aim for one gram of omega-3s per day. The American Heart Association recommends up to 3 grams of omega-3s per day to lower triglycerides.
- Consume a GLA supplement, for example borage oil, to ensure proper levels of the anti-inflammatory omega-6.
- Flax seeds are the best sources of omega-3s in the plant kingdom.
- Eat walnuts, Brazil nuts, butter nuts, macadamia nuts.
- The more green, the better. Dark green leafy vegetables are good sources of omega-3s. Try

romaine lettuce, mixed greens, spirulina, purslane, kale, Swiss chard, and arugula.

- Make your own salad dressing using flax oil.
- Avoid refined grocery store oils. These oils are heavily processed and contain an abundance of unhealthy omega-6s, which can lead to insulin resistance. Use extra virgin olive oil, coconut oil, and macadamia nut oil as your primary cooking oils.
- To shed unwanted belly fat, use a high linoleic acid safflower oil as a daily supplement (see Chapter 8 on SafSlim™).
- When possible, consume free-range meat, which contains higher levels of omega-3s than grain-fed meat. The grain fed to the animals is rich in pro-inflammatory omega-6s, which changes the fatty acid profile of the meat and leads to fat imbalances.

CHAPTER 4

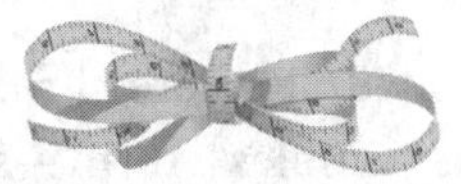

Belly-Safe Carbohydrates

Just like the wrong types of fat in our diet contribute to belly fat, so too do the wrong types of carbohydrates. The low-fat diet craze reigned supreme throughout the late 1980s and early 1990s during which fat-free or low-fat food items were the way to help you shed those unwanted pounds. However, people didn't realize that by eating a low-fat diet, they were actually replacing those fat calories with sugar, also known as refined carbohydrates. Did the low-fat diets make us any thinner? No!!! In fact, we saw belly fat increase and obesity rates skyrocket, leading us to believe that perhaps it isn't fat that makes us fat but that sugar and other carbohydrates may have more to do with it.

Why do our bodies have such a difficult time adjusting to sugar and other carbohydrate foods? The carbohydrates we eat today are modern-day foods that have led to modern-day diseases. In this chapter, we are going to learn how to distinguish between the good carbohydrates and the bad carbohydrates, choosing those that our body can recognize, which will help prevent excess belly fat and insulin resistance.

GOOD CARBS, BETTER CARBS

Digestible carbohydrates are broken down in the intestine into their simplest form—sugar—which then enters the blood. As blood sugar levels rise, special cells in the pancreas churn out more and more insulin. To reduce high sugar levels, the pancreas secretes large amounts of insulin, which helps transport the sugar from your food into cells where it is burned for energy (chiefly in muscle cells) or stored as glycogen (in the liver) or fat (in adipose cells). As cells sponge up blood sugar, sugar levels in the bloodstream fall back to a preset minimum, as do insulin levels. Over time, when you have continually high levels of sugar, insulin levels must remain high to deal with the excess sugar; however, elevated insulin levels overwhelm the limited number of insulin cell receptors that our body has. Thus, in essence, these elevated sugar levels stress out our insulin receptors, making them resistant to insulin.

Insulin resistance causes both blood sugar and insulin levels to remain high long after eating. Over time, the heavy demands put on the insulin-making cells wears them out, and insulin production slows and then stops. Genes, a sedentary lifestyle, belly fat, and eating a diet filled with foods that cause big spikes in blood sugar can all promote insulin resistance.

FIX IT WITH FIBER – THE IMPORTANCE OF DIETARY FIBER

Eating lots of fiber-rich foods is one of the simplest and easiest things you can do to shrink you belly. Fiber gives your metabolism a boost and keeps you feeling full so you don't overeat, and fortunately, it's pretty easy to get more fiber into your diet. Simply start buying "whole grain" versions of your favorite foods, including breads, cereals, and pastas. Eat more dishes made with beans and legumes. Learn to incorporate a variety of fiber-rich fruits and vegetables into your recipes—both the fresh and frozen versions are great.Today, we live in a fiber-deficient society. The majority of North Americans consume only one-quarter to one-half of the Institute of Medicine's recommended fiber levels of 38 grams per day for men and 25 grams per day for women. In fact, the average daily fiber intake is only 12 grams for women and 18 grams for men.

Types of Fiber

There are two main types of fiber that are important for health: soluble and insoluble. Soluble fiber is found in flaxseed, oats, barley, and legumes and in smaller amounts in fruits and vegetables. Soluble fiber forms a gelatin-like substance and works to increase the water content of the stool. Soluble fibers acts like a sponge, binding excess toxins, blood cholesterol, and blood sugar and is an important nutrient for the dietary management of high cholesterol and diabetes.

Insoluble fiber is found in flaxseeds, wheat, bran, and whole grains and in smaller amounts in fruits and vegetables. Insoluble fiber sweeps the colon, increases stool size, and helps relieve constipation and gas. Research also shows that consuming sufficient amounts of insoluble fiber plays an important role in satiety (the feeling of fullness) and may help people lose weight. Not surprisingly, excess belly fat and obesity is less prevalent in populations that consume a high-fiber diet.

Sources of Fiber

SOLUBLE FIBER	INSOLUBLE FIBER
Oatmeal	Whole grains, such as whole-wheat breads, barley, couscous, brown rice, and bulgur
Oatbran	Whole-grain breakfast cereals
Nuts and seeds	Wheat bran
Legumes, such as dried peas, beans, and lentils	Seeds
Apples	Carrots
Pears	Cucumbers
Strawberries	Zucchini
Blueberries	Celery
Sweet Potatoes	Tomatoes

There are numerous benefits to consuming fiber. A high-fiber diet will promote increased chewing and slower eating, delay gastric emptying (keeping you feeling full longer—up to 4 hours post meal), stabilize blood sugar levels, absorb toxins, reduce cholesterol in your blood, increase stool size, and reduce your overall risk of chronic disease.

Fiber Beats Belly Fat

A high-fiber diet will help you get rid of belly fat and promotes great health. The fact is, people on a high-fiber diet will be able to manage their weight and health much more easily than people who aren't eating enough fiber. Why?

- Fiber helps to curb your appetite. A high-fiber diet helps to regulate your blood glucose levels by slowing down the time it takes for food to leave the stomach and by delaying the absorption of glucose (blood sugar) from a meal. Eating fiber-rich foods keeps you full longer and helps control your hunger—all of which are beneficial for getting lean.
- Fiber reduces the absorption of calories because it is indigestible but has no fattening calories. Fiber acts as a blocking agent that stops the absorption of calories consumed and flushes calories out of the body. In other words, it gets rid of the calories you eat. Remember this calculation: for every gram of fiber you eat, you can eliminate up to 7 calories from your diet. So, if you are eating the recommended level of

25-38 grams, you can subtract 175-266 calories from your diet each day. This alone will help you lose 0.5 to 1 pound per week.

- Fiber-rich foods typically contain fewer calories; therefore, you can eat a lot of food without eating a lot of calories.
- Fiber-rich foods help increase insulin sensitivity: the more sensitive your cells are to insulin, the less fat will be deposited in the belly.

Fiber-Rich Foods for a Lean Belly

- Start the day with whole grains. If you're partial to hot cereals, try old-fashioned or steel-cut oats or barley.
- Use whole-grain breads for lunch or snacks. Check the label to make sure the whole wheat or other whole grain is the first ingredient listed.
- Experiment with beans, legumes, and lentils by including them in various dishes, such as chili, soups, and salad.
- Limit the amount of processed, refined, and starchy foods you eat, as they tend to be lower in fiber.
- Eat unlimited amounts of vegetables. Most veggies are so low in carbohydrates that they have no measurable effect on blood sugar levels. Vegetables, such as tomatoes, lettuce, cucumbers, peppers, and

onions, can be considered "free foods," as even in large amounts, they have no effect on blood sugar levels.

CHAPTER 5

Protein-Packed Belly

Fiber-rich carbohydrates, healthy fats, and protein are all important for preventing and dealing with excess belly fat. Now that we have discussed carbohydrates and healthy fats, it is time to examine your diet and see if you are eating sufficient amounts of protein. Protein is the only nutrient that causes the body to build muscle, which helps supercharge your metabolism for fat loss. Remember a tight tummy is made in the kitchen, not the gym.

We must be aware of the types of proteins that are consumed in the United States, keeping in mind the way we feed our livestock. The shift from consuming grass-fed meat sources to grain-fed sources has resulted in poorer quality meat that is higher in the pro-inflammatory types of fat that are linked to belly fat.

This is why you need to be very careful about choosing high-quality protein sources in your diet and should consume a high-quality protein at each meal and with each snack. Balancing protein with fibrous carbohydrates and healthy monounsaturated and polyunsaturated fats is the key to preventing belly fat and getting rid of it if it has already made its way to your waistline. Let's recall what we have already discussed for the food/belly fat connection:

- Decrease saturated and trans fats.
- Incorporate more essential fatty acids from nuts, seeds, fatty fish, and green leafy vegetables as well as the healthy omega-9 fats from olive oil and avocadoes.
- Decrease your consumption of refined carbohydrates, including white sugar, white rice, and white pasta.
- Increase your consumption of fiber-rich carbohydrates.
- Choose high-quality proteins and balance protein foods at snack and meal times.

Combining proteins with fiber-rich carbohydrates is essential to help balance the effects on your blood glucose and insulin levels. It also helps keep you feeling full and aids in developing and maintaining muscle. In addition, protein is needed to build your body (hair, nails, bone matrix, cell membranes, enzymes, etc.), and from a weight-control perspective, it helps curb your appetite. Adequate protein intake also means you are eating less fat and fewer carbohydrates.

If you aren't eating enough protein, your body can't perform all the functions for which it is required. Over time, you may feel tired and sluggish and be more susceptible to illness, and if you fail to build muscle, your chances of developing insulin resistance and belly fat increase.

BALANCING PROTEIN

So how much protein does one really need to consume? My preference, as I mentioned before, is to consume a protein food every time you eat.

Typically, the recommended daily requirement for protein for adults is 50-70 grams of protein per day (depending on if you're female or male). If you are very physically active and/or trying to lose weight, you may want to increase your consumption of protein up to higher levels (i.e.,1 gram/kg body weight). Your overall aim for your food choices should be about 15-20% of your calories from protein, 45-50% from fiber-rich carbohydrates, and no more than 25-30% from fat (remember to focus on the mono- and polyunsaturated fats).

You are probably wondering how you can tell how much protein you are eating at each meal. Three to seven servings of meat, dairy, fish, and meat alternatives, such as legumes and beans, is a good start.

The Whey It Is

Many of you will have difficulty consuming the recommended levels of high-quality protein through diet alone. Meeting these protein requirements is difficult despite the fact that most North Americans get plenty of protein; the problem is the protein-laden foods we generally consume are associated with high levels of fat and cholesterol. As such, one of the nutrition products I include in my own personal nutrition regime is the use of whey protein. Whey protein is a naturally complete protein, meaning that it contains all of the essential amino acids required in your daily diet. Further, high-quality whey protein has been shown in the scientific data to promote fat loss and is a great way to meet your protein requirements.

For example, you could have two whey protein shakes per day and then combine them with three smaller meals: drink one protein shake mid-morning (containing 20-25 grams of whey protein) and another an hour before dinner, both of which will control your appetite at common craving times. I love making power protein smoothies in the morning in my blender. It's a great way to start the day and jumpstart your metabolism. See my recipe below.

Flax Berry Blast

1 scoop (25 grams) whey protein isolate
1 cup berries (fresh or frozen)
1 tbsp ground flaxseeds
1 tsp organic flax oil
1 cup milk beverage or water
To Prepare: Mix in blender and enjoy

Whey to Weight Loss

A diet based on increased, but not excessive levels of protein, has been shown in a number of studies to give an added boost to dieters by helping them increase weight loss, increase body fat loss, and reduce muscle tissue loss. The body requires more energy to digest protein than other foods; as a result, you burn more calories after a protein meal. In addition, recent studies have highlighted the role of the essential amino acid leucine in improving body composition. High-quality whey protein is rich in leucine and thus helps preserve lean muscle tissue while promoting fat loss. Further, this amino acid works with insulin to stimulate protein synthesis in muscle. In fact, whey protein contains more leucine than milk protein, egg protein, and soy protein.

Whey protein also contains components that help stimulate the release of two appetite-suppressing hormones: cholecystokinin (CCK) and glucagon-like peptide (GLP)

Whey Protein & Ingredient Labels

To make sure you are getting the important benefits of whey protein, always check the ingredient label before you buy a product. One of the following should be listed as the first or second ingredient on the label:

- *Whey protein isolate*
- *Whey protein concentrate*

If the ingredient label contains any of the following statements, check further to be sure the product has an acceptable amount of whey protein.

- *Protein Blend: Whey proteins may or may not be an ingredient. If they are part of the protein blend, you have no way of knowing what the concentration level is.*
- *Hydrolyzed Protein: The protein in this product may be a protein of lesser quality, such as gelatin protein.*

Protein Your Way

Overall, total protein intake should not be excessive and should be reasonably proportional to the carbohydrates and fat you consume daily. The selected protein foods should be a mixture of high-quality animal proteins (eggs, chicken, turkey, etc.), plant proteins, and whey protein supplements, so as not to provide excess total fat, saturated fat, or cholesterol.

CHAPTER 6

Getting It All Started

It's surprising how most of us don't really know what to eat or even where to start. Did you ever wonder why there are so many fad diets out there? It's because people are desperate to figure out what to eat. Fad diets are a multibillion dollar industry in which products are marketed to consumers with magical claims. In many cases, once you go off the diet, not only do you regain the weight lost, but you add some extra as well. The diet industry's success is built on our failures.

But why didn't these fad diets help you lose weight or keep the weight off? Fad diets are generally so unrealistic and so unpleasant that they cannot be maintained for the long term. Most of us who try a fad diet will stop following the diet because it's too restrictive, boring, and expensive, and is an overall stressful experience. A recent study published in the *Annals of Internal Medicine* showed there is little evidence to support the use of many commercial weight-loss programs.

Healthy eating is about maintaining a balanced diet to ensure that you are getting all of the nutrients your body needs. This means consuming an assortment of foods in the right amounts from all of the food groups. A proper combination of these foods will ensure that your metabolism and appetite remain in a healthy state.

The eating plan I have designed is based on teaching you about healthy eating and making the proper food choices because a lasting change in your eating habits and activity level will result in weight loss and eventually maintaining a healthy weight.

Fat Burning Foods

There are foods that have been shown to burn fat and keep your metabolism revved up. The goal is to eat foods that burn more calories than the food itself, which, in turn, will help your body burn stored fat. Here is a quick check list of foods you can incorporate into your daily diet to help burn belly fat:

- Calcium-rich dairy products, including milk, cheese, and plain/natural yogurt, are rich in calcium, which research has shown can boost fat loss by increasing the breakdown of fat cells. Scientists have discovered that eating three servings of dairy products per day helped overweight people lose more belly fat than those on a similar diet minus the dairy. If you are lactose intolerant (that is, you have difficulty digesting the sugar in milk) use Lactaid or enzymes that are beneficial for breaking down milk sugars.

- Nuts, which are rich in protein and healthy mono- and polyunsaturated fats, help keep you feeling full, increase leptin levels and increase your body's ability to burn fat.
- Protein foods are essential in burning belly fat.
- Fiber-rich foods help stabilize blood sugar levels, keep your tummy feeling full, curb appetite, improve digestion, and help banish belly fat.
- Green tea helps speed up your metabolism and assists your body in burning more fat than carbohydrates for energy, which will help shed dangerous belly fat. Drink several cups per day.
- Apples contain pectin, which is thought to restrict cells from absorbing fat. Pectin also encourages water absorption from food, which helps break up fat deposits.
- Healthy fats like omega-3s from fish oil help improve the cells ability to burn fat more efficiently. Incorporate 1000 mg of omega-3 in supplement form into your daily routine.
- Emulsified high linoleic acid safflower oil has been shown in university-level studies to assist in targeted belly fat loss by improving adiponectin levels. At the same time safflower oil helps to improve lean muscle mass and balance blood sugar.

- Chilies or cayenne pepper contain capsaicin, which increases metabolism. Because these types of pepper are thermogenic, they will help the body burn extra calories after eating.
- Eat your greens. Veggies are broken down slowly in the body, causing less of a rise in blood sugar levels, less insulin secretion, and, ultimately, less fat storage. Vegetables also have high water and fiber content, which helps promote the feeling of fullness, reduces hunger, and decreases calorie intake.
- Drink plenty of water to help keep your cells hydrated, your metabolism revved, and your tummy feeling full.

Taking Stock

To discover more about your food and activity habits, answer the following questions:

1. Do you eat fish and poultry at least three times a week?
   ❑ No ❑ Yes
2. Do you eat breakfast every day?
   ❑ No ❑ Yes
3. Do you eat whole grains instead of white or refined grains?
   ❑ No ❑ Yes

4. Do you eat low-fat dairy products whenever you can?
   ❑ No ❑ Yes
5. Do you avoid all fried foods as much as possible?
   ❑ No ❑ Yes
6. Do you eat three to five meals per day?
   ❑ No ❑ Yes
7. Do you eat fast food less than once a week?
   ❑ No ❑ Yes
8. Do you pay attention to portion sizes?
   ❑ No ❑ Yes
9. Do you follow a healthy eating plan and avoid going on and off diets?
   ❑ No ❑ Yes
10. Do you set aside at least 30 minutes three times a week for physical activity?
    ❑ No ❑ Yes

Your Score: Count up the number of checks you have in column 2 (yes). What was your score? ___

- 8-10 checks: Fantastic! Keep up the good work.
- 5-7 checks: You're on the right track, but it's time to start considering some changes.
- 0-4 checks: Uh-oh. Take time now to make some changes.

Tell Me How

In the beginning, the changes you make may be as simple as making the switch from white bread to whole-grain bread; from margarine to butter; from eating hamburgers two times per week to eating chicken, turkey, and other leaner cuts of meat. If you have been consuming a poor diet for a number of years and have belly fat and the changes you need to make will not happen overnight. Remember, it has taken a lifetime to get to this weight; it will take some time to get your waistline back to a healthy weight. Setting reasonable goals for yourself will be the key to successful weight loss.

A diet to beat belly fat aims at improving insulin sensitivity. Food changes should focus on fat loss, which will improve insulin sensitivity. Research has shown that in most cases, a 5-10% weight reduction is sufficient to see significant improvement in insulin resistance.

So how do we start eating right to improve our insulin resistance, lose belly fat, and improve our overall health? Listed below are the food recommendations for optimal health:

- Vegetables (five to seven servings per day): Choose green foods more often. Start lunch and dinner with a green salad.
- Protein (five to six servings per day or each time you eat): Lean meat, chicken, turkey, fish, eggs, lentils, and whey protein. Eat protein at each meal

to balance blood sugar levels. Remember, protein and fiber-rich carbohydrates should be consumed together.

- Healthy Fats (four to five servings per day): Nuts, seeds, avocadoes, fatty fish, and oils (e.g., flax seed oil, extra virgin olive oil, macadamia nut oil, butter, and coconut oil).
- Whole Grains (three to five servings per day): Fiber-rich choices only. Increase fiber consumption to 25 to 30 grams per day. Limit your carbohydrate consumption to what you can actually burn because what you don't burn will be stored as fat.
- Dairy (two to four servings per day): Choose low-fat organic dairy foods more often. Try incorporating yogurt, cottage cheese, and kefir into your diet. These choices are even better than milk because of their beneficial bacteria.
- Fruit (two to three servings): Of the two to three servings, you should be consuming at least one serving of berries.

Here are some other recommendations to get your health back on track:

- Consume a diet rich in whole raw foods that have gone through minimal processing.
- Reduce calorie consumption by 500 calories per day

to safely lose one pound per week. Combine fewer calories with burning an additional 500 calories per day during exercise, and you can lose two pounds per week.

- Eat five to six small meals per day. If you are in the initial phases of weight loss, you may want to consider replacing one or two meals per day with a whey protein shake.
- Never skip breakfast. Your mom was right; breakfast is the most important meal of the day. Having protein at breakfast helps to jump start your metabolism.
- Avoid starchy or sugary foods—get rid of everything white in your cupboards.
- Avoid hydrogenated oils (trans fats) and junk foods (high-calorie, low-nutrient foods).
- Utilize whey protein powders to help stabilize blood sugar levels.
- Eliminate artificial sweeteners; switch to natural sweeteners like stevia and xylitol.
- Limit salt intake.
- Limit alcohol consumption.
- Try to exercise daily—try to burn 250 to 500 calories per day.
- Drink lots of water—eight glasses per day.

- Supplement with a whole food multivitamin and omega-3 fish oil every day. If you are overweight or if you have insulin resistance, excess belly fat, type 2 diabetes, or cardiovascular disease, add in SafSlim™ to help improve adiponectin levels and decrease belly fat.
- Get plenty of sleep. Scientific studies increasingly link lack of sleep to the obesity epidemic.

Eat More Frequently

Eating five to six smaller meals per day is highly recommended. I recommend breakfast, a protein shake mid-morning, lunch, a protein shake mid-afternoon, dinner, and then an optional snack in the evening. This eating schedule helps balance blood sugar levels, keeping them even throughout the day, and will prevent spikes and dips in blood sugar and insulin levels.

Meal Plans and Meal Replacements

As mentioned earlier, if you are in the beginning phases of weight loss, you may want to consider substituting one or two meals a day with a protein shake. In between the protein shakes, you can have snacks containing protein, fiber-rich carbohydrates, vegetables, or berries. Thus, instead of drinking a protein shake between meals, you would use it to replace a meal.

Taking Action

Set realistic goals so you can be confident that you will be able to keep this commitment to yourself. Review your responses to the "Taking Stock" quiz and think of small changes that will help you achieve a healthier lifestyle. Eating an extra piece of fruit a day instead of a dessert, weeding the garden, or walking to the shop are easy ways to introduce lifestyle improvements.

My eating goals include the following:

1. ____

2. ____

3. ____

CHAPTER 7

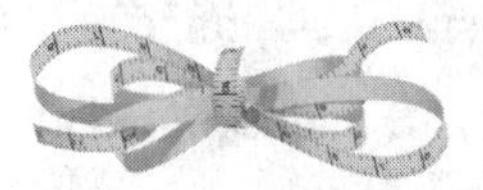

Fitness for a Lean Belly

Fitness Contributor: Ingrid Vadina

This is my favorite chapter because I was able to enlist the help of my trainer, Ingrid Vadina. She has years of experience as a personal trainer and has helped thousands of clients successfully meet their physical activity goals. I hired Ingrid after I had my first son to help regain strength in my core. We quickly became friends, as I love surrounding myself with like-minded individuals who are healthy, positive, and can motivate others to achieve their personal best. I have always been amazed with Ingrid, especially for her discipline when training for fitness competitions. Her workout in this chapter is highly effective, fun, and targets belly fat spot on.

Benefits of Regular Exercise

Increasing your physical activity will have dramatic benefits on your health:

- Decreases insulin resistance and can aid in both preventing type 2 diabetes and cardiovascular disease and managing metabolic syndrome.

- Helps your body burn calories to help you lose weight.
- Increases insulin resistance.
- Helps build and maintain healthy bones, muscles, and joints.
- Decreases body fat, especially belly fat.
- Increases serotonin levels (the feel-good, happy hormone).
- Gives you a positive outlook on life.
- Improves sleep.
- Helps control stress levels.

Importance of Strength Training

Cardiovascular activity has many benefits for heart health, it releases endorphins that give you a sense of euphoria and wellbeing, and it will help you burn calories; however, it will not reshape your body. Your muscles will not get tight by doing cardio only! So what will help you reshape your body? Strength training.

Regular resistance training will increase your muscle, which is essential for weight loss because muscle is very active tissue with high-energy requirements for maintenance. In fact, it burns more calories than any other body tissue.

Remember this:

- Every pound of muscle burns between 40 to 120 calories per day just to sustain itself.

- Every pound of fat burns between 1 to 3 calories to sustain itself.

Regular weight training combined with cardiovascular activity and eating five to six small meals per day will turn your body into a fat-burning machine even when you sleep. The more muscle you have, the faster your metabolism is, which means the more weight you will lose. Your metabolism is a direct reflection of the lifestyle choices you make.

In addition, most adults experience a decrease of approximately 5-7 pounds of muscle tissue per decade. Thus, strength training is important for preventing muscle loss that normally accompanies the aging process. We lose up to one-half pound of muscle every year after age 25 unless we perform regular strength exercise.

A Strong Core for a Lean Belly

Having a strong core is more beneficial than you might think. A solid core protects your lower back, improves your balance, and provides postural stability. When you keep your abdominal muscles contracted, you work on your core all day long.

Because it is difficult to spot reduce with exercise, the best way to start is to work your full body. To lose fat in your belly, you need to decrease your total body fat. Often I hear my clients tell me that they keep doing sit ups and crunches and they don't see any results in their bellies. Please keep in mind that an endless amount of crunches will not get you any closer to your goal of having a flatter stomach, but full-body workouts will. Overtraining your abdominals is actually one of the most common mistakes made by beginners in the gym.

How Much Weight Will I Lose?

Of course everyone wants to experience those success stories they see on TV of people losing 50 to 100 pounds; however, it is important to set realistic and healthy goals. Aim for 0.5-2 pounds of fat loss per week.

Although some people may lose 3-5 pounds for the first two weeks, losing more than 1-2 pounds per week after generally means that you are losing muscle mass and will lead to a lower metabolic rate and decreased energy. Losing weight quickly may also contribute to excess skin, so a slow and steady approach to fat loss is always your best bet.

For others, it might take longer for your metabolism to kick in. In fact, it might take several weeks to lose even 1 pound. Remember your water can fluctuate in one day up to around 6 pounds.

Motivation Is Key

You can have the best plan in the world, but if you do not have the internal motivation, it will be difficult to stick to your new healthy routine. Here is a quick summary of things to keep in mind when starting an exercise program:

- Put your health on top of your priority list. There will always be something else to do if you let things get in your way.
- Set REALISTIC short- and long-term goals and visualize your success. I suggest setting weekly and monthly goals.
- Spend 5-10 minutes at the end of each week going through your schedule and figuring out ways to fit in exercise for the next week.
- Put target dates on your goals and stick to them.
- Keep a journal of your workouts.
- Schedule motivational time into your daily routine.
- Surround yourself with positive people who will support you in reaching your goals.
- Find balance in your life. For instance, getting enough sleep and having time to relax is very important.

Get Me Started

For anyone who currently does no activity, starting even moderate amounts of regular physical activity may be difficult. Your daily physical activity target should be built up in small activity "portions" (10-15 minutes) over time. Your rate of progression will depend on several factors, including age, functional capacity, medical status, personal preferences, and goals.

Check Your Posture

Proper postural alignment is the key to looking younger and thinner as well as to improving your health and wellbeing. When your back is in a neutral spine alignment, the ligaments, muscles, and discs are at their optimal position and are under the least amount of stress. Think of a string pulling from the top of your head elongating your spine. Aim to maintain a neutral spine during daily activities and exercise, as maintaining proper posture will reduce your chances of injury and maximize your exercise benefits. In addition, proper alignment can improve your breathing and increase your confidence.

Resistance Training

Proper form and technique will significantly increase the efficiency of your workouts and reduce your risk of injury. The most common mistake I see around the gym is using wrong technique, having improper form, swinging weights, using too much weight, and doing too much too soon. When this happens, it is likely that your muscles aren't actually getting any significant workout at all, certainly not an effective one. Mastering proper form and technique before you increase your resistance is crucial.

During every exercise, keep your core tight and back straight, making sure not to arch in order to complete the exercise. Avoid locking your knees and your elbows. Keep your head in line with your spine, and keep your wrists straight while holding weights or bands.

Avoid Holding Your Breath

It is very important that you avoid holding your breath during your workouts. When you hold your breath, the amount of oxygen getting to the muscles and brain becomes limited, while blood pressure and heart rate increase to extreme levels. Lifting heavy weight while holding your breath could cause dizziness, fainting, and—in extreme cases—hernias or even heart attacks. To breathe correctly, exhale during exertion (the lifting portion of the exercise) and inhale during the lowering phase of an exercise.

Speed of Movement

Make a conscious effort to lift at a certain speed. For beginners counting 2 seconds up and 2 seconds down for each repetition encourages good movement patterns.

Avoid using momentum, as it puts unnecessary stress on your joints and will not give you the full benefits of an exercise; make your muscles do the work, not gravity.

Sets and Repetitions

What is a set? This term refers to repeating the same exercise a certain number of times. For example doing ten push ups could be one set of that exercise.

What is a repetition? This refers to the number of times you perform an exercise during a set. Ten push ups means ten repetitions.

Change your workout

Remember the secret to successful resistance training is to constantly challenge your muscles by increasing either the resistance level, doing more repetitions, incorporating more sets. Additionally, your muscles need a break in order to properly respond to exercises. Avoid training the same muscle groups day after day. You need to have at least a 48-hour break between working out the same muscle groups. Further, you should usually change your program completely every four to eight weeks.

Warm Up and Cool Down

Each exercise session should incorporate a five- to ten-minute pre-exercise warm up and a five- to ten-minute post-exercise cool down of low-intensity aerobic exercise (walking, cycling, etc.) or slow rhythmic stretching exercises to prevent injuries. Depending on your level of physical conditioning, physical activity longer than 30 minutes is encouraged as tolerated.

The purpose of the warm up is to increase your body temperature and heart rate to slowly prepare your body for the workout. Walking, cycling, rowing, kickbacks, knee ups, and step ups are few ways to warm up. Active dynamic stretches are also recommended to take your joints through their range of motion before putting more strain on them. Movements like arm rotations, spinal rotations, extensions, and some lateral movements are great ways to move your joints.

After cardio activity, you will need to return your body and heart rate to its pre-exercise state, which will reduce the chance of post-exercise light-headedness or fainting. To cool down your body, perform the activity you were doing before working out (e.g., if you were walking fast to warm up, cool down by walking slowly). Stretching is also a great form of cool down.

CARDIO

Before starting a cardio workout, you need to determine the level of your intensity. RPE (Rate of Perceived Exertion) and the talk test are methods for determining your aerobic exercise intensity without using your age and resting heart rate.

RPE

Simply rate the activity on scale of 1-10 with 1 being very easy and 10 being maximum intensity. This method works for many people, as heart rate monitoring may not reflect accurate intensity for many people taking certain medications or those with genetic/trained low heart rates.

Talk Test

I love using this method for beginners. I make sure my clients can comfortably carry on a conversation during their workout. Once they experience shortness of breath, I decrease the intensity

- Level 1: Very easy—Seated and relaxing
- Level 5: Above moderate—Breathing moderately hard but can still talk
- Level 10: Maximal—Can't maintain and must stop after a period of time

HR Max

To calculate your exercise heart rate using your age, use this formula:

(Training %) x (220-Age) = Training Heart Rate

So, for example, if you are 30 years old and you need to keep your HR between 60-70% of your HR Max, your exercise heart rate should be between 114 and 133 beats per minute.

Determine Your Exercise Heart Rate

You can locate your carotid pulse during an exercise by lightly pressing one or two fingers in the hollow of your neck below the back corner of your jaw.

Do not use your thumb, as it has a pulse of its own, and do not press too hard because that can slow blood flow. Count the number of beats in 10 seconds and multiply by six.

A Word on Cardio

People who are new to fitness, haven't been exercising for a long time, and are leading sedentary lifestyle are **beginners** to fitness.

I recommend starting cardio with any enjoyable activity—anything you will be able to stick with. Walking, cycling, dancing, swimming, taking your kids for a walk—these are all great ways to start. Even just using stairs instead of the elevator or parking your car farther from the store will make a big difference for an unconditioned person. Start with as low as 5-15 minutes three times a week, and if you cannot sustain that activity, perform shorter bouts of cardio training several times per day.

Remember, beginners should choose an intensity during which they can comfortably talk but are breathing heavier than usually. Using the talk test is great way to determine your level of intensity. If you feel you are out of your breath, slow down.

Intermediate people are those who are comfortably able to sustain 30 minutes of cardio activity and are doing so three to five times per week on a regular basis.

I recommend you start increasing your intensity at this time. You are safe to go up to 85% of your heart rate maximum. Interval training, like the circuit below, is designed for intermediate-level participants to keep their heart rate higher.

Your Cardio Workout Plan

- Very unconditioned individuals: 5-15 minutes three times per week.
    - Intensity: RPE (1-2), 50-60% HR Max, very easy, you are able to talk comfortably
- Beginners: 15-30 minutes three to five times per week.
    - Intensity: RPE (2-3), 60-70% HR Max, you are breathing heavier but are able talk comfortably
- Intermediate: 30 – 45 minutes, three to five times per week;
    - Intensity: RPE (3-5), 65-75% HR Max, fill this out.

There are many different ways to train effectively. The workout below can be done anywhere: in your living room, backyard, or hotel room. All you need is resistance bands, a timer, a pedometer, a towel, and a bottle of water. Isn't it great? No more excuses!

WHAT IS CIRCUIT TRAINING?

This workout is designed in the form of circuit and is highly effective for fat loss and general conditioning. You control intensity by increasing/decreasing breaks between exercises, the duration of cardio exercises, the number of repetitions, breaks between sets, and the amount of exercises you perform. This is why this workout is effective for participants with different fitness levels. The goal for beginners in this circuit is to keep your heart rate at a comfortable level—that means being able to carry on a conversation. Intermediate participants will keep their intensity at a level where it is difficult to talk.

Circuit Program–Beginners

If you are beginner, this program will keep your heart rate up while burning more calories.

You will exercise all major muscle groups in one continuous cycle.

Perform two to three times a week, one to two sets of 15 repetitions. You will perform 15-30 seconds of cardio-type exercises in between the resistance training exercises. Follow up to 12 weeks.

Intermediate

In this program, intermediate participants will mostly increase their muscular endurance and cardiovascular fitness. If you are doing cardio regularly but have never done resistance training exercises before, follow the circuit training for beginners.

Increase intensity for jumping jacks, knee ups, and kickbacks. Perform all 12 exercises and change your program after four to eight weeks.

As you progress you can make this workout more challenging by having no breaks between exercises and increasing your sets.

CIRCUIT TRAINING PROGRAM

Perform three times a week with moderate intensity, two to three sets, between 15-20 repetitions. The correct weight should produce fatigue at the last repetition.
(This circuit is a combination of weight-bearing exercise and short bouts of cardio activity)

WARM UP: Perform 5 minutes of activities like knee ups, kickbacks, marching in place, side-to-side steps, or step ups. Listen to your body, and make sure you are warm before you start the circuit. Perform activities that include ROM moves like, arm rotation.

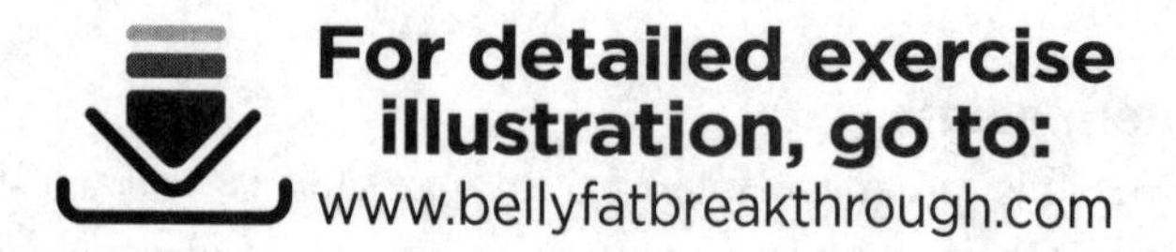

1. SEATED ROW

EASIER VERSION: Sitting on the floor, your legs is in front of you slightly bent. Your band is wrapped up around your feet and you are holding the tubes with your hands, keeping elbows close to your body. Make sure your resistance is not too hard or not to easy to perform your repetitions. Keep your back straight and pull handles towards your body. Squeeze your shoulder blades. Hold for a second and return slowly.

HARDER VERSION: Increase your tension by wrapping the tubing twice around your legs or choose stronger tubing.

MUSCLE WORKED: Back and bicep (latissimus dorsi, rhomboids, trapezius, and bicep brachii)

2. CARDIO–JUMPING JACKS

EASIER VERSION: Low-impact jumping jacks (moving legs to the side one at the time

HARDER VERSION: Stand with your hands by your size and then in an explosive movement, jump directly up, moving both legs out to the side and arms up above shoulder.

3. PUSH UPS

EASIER VERSION: Push ups against the wall or push ups on your knees.

- Wall push ups—stand arms-length away from a wall, place your hands on the wall, arms shoulder width apart, and perform a vertical push up.
- Knee push ups—Lie face down with your arms straight, your palms flat on the floor, your hands shoulder width apart, knees on the floor (keeping shoulders, hips, and knees in line). Bend your elbows to bring your torso near the floor, avoid arching your back. Push yourself back to an arms-extended position.

HARDER VERSION: Regular push ups performed with feet on the floor slightly apart.

MUSCLE WORKED: Chest, front shoulders, and triceps (pectoralis major, anterior deltoids, tricep brachii)

4. CARDIO–PRETEND SKIPPING

EASIER VERSION: As easy as lifting legs/jogging in place with forearms rotating

HARDER VERSION: Skip with your feet together and forearms rotating.

Beginner Duration: 15-30 seconds
Intermediate Duration: 30 seconds

5. UPRIGHT ROW

EASIER VERSION: Stand out straight with your knees soft. Secure the center of the band under the arches of your feet and grip the handles with your hands facing out and close together. Pull the handles up to chest level with elbows out to the side and slightly above your shoulder, then slowly return to the starting position.

HARDER VERSION: Increase your tension by keeping your legs farther apart or choosing stronger tubing

MUSCLE WORKED: Upper back and shoulders (trapezius, deltoids)

6. CARDIO–KICKBACKS

EASIER VERSION: Bring your heels up behind you one leg at the time, and try to kick yourself in the butt.

HARDER VERSION: Stay on your toes for the entire duration of the move.

Duration: 15-30 seconds

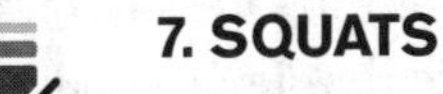

7. SQUATS

EASIER VERSION: Wall squats, and Chair squats

- **Wall Squats:** Practice proper technique facing the wall. Stand 2 inches in front of the wall (facing the wall), your feet shoulder width apart, lower hips until your thighs are parallel to the floor. Avoid touching your face, chest, and knees to the wall while keeping your back straight and not rounding your buttocks or arching. Once you are able to master this you can perform regular squats.

- **Chair squats:** People who a have hard time performing squats can start with seated chair squats. Your knees should be levelled or slightly higher than your hips. Avoid taking your knees past your toes.

HARDER VERSION: (Regular squats) Position your feet shoulder width apart, lower your hips until your thighs are parallel to the floor. Avoid leaning forward and rounding your back, and avoid taking your knees past your toes. Remember your form from the wall squats. Resistance can be also added

MUSCLE WORKED: Legs (hamstrings, quadriceps, gluteus maximus)

8. CARDIO–SKATE/SIDE-TO-SIDE (LATERAL JUMPS)

EASIER VERSION: From standing, take a step to the side, then bring your other leg across to meet it. One leg stays on the ground. Do the same movement to the opposite side.

HARDER VERSION: Make steps are longer and don't let either leg touch the ground for very long.
Duration: 15-30 seconds

9. ABDOMINAL CRUNCH

EASIER VERSION: Lie on your back with your legs together, knees bent, and feet flat on the floor. Tighten your stomach muscles and slowly lift your head and upper back off the floor without activating your hip muscles. Press lower back to the floor. For an even easier version, you can place your arms across the chest or on your thighs. Hold on top for 1 second and slowly return back to the floor. Keep your head in line with your spine.

HARDER VERSION: Keep your hands behind your head but avoid pulling your head with your hands. Hold your abs tight for 2 seconds in the up position and 1 second in down position without touching the floor with your head and keeping constant tension in your abs. Avoid using hip flexors. Press lower back to the floor.

MUSCLE WORKED: Abs (rectus abdominals, external obliques, internal obliques)

10. TABLE TOPS

Kneeling down, keep your hands exactly under your shoulders and your knees under your hips. Keep your back straight. Extend your right leg to the level of your hip and your left arm to the level of your shoulder. Hold for 2 seconds and switch sides. Avoid arching your back.

MUSCLE WORKED: Lower back, middle back, buttocks, and rear shoulder (erector spinae, lower trapezius, posterior deltoids)

11. BICEP CURLS

EASIER VERSION: Hold band at each end, making sure you create the same resistance by stepping onto the middle of the band with your foot.Your palms should be facing forward. Bend your elbows, raising the weight up toward your shoulders without moving your elbows. Squeeze your bicep muscle and return slowly to the starting position. Avoid swinging your arms and moving/arching your back.

HARDER VERSION: Increase your tension by placing your feet slightly apart or choosing stronger tubing.

MUSCLE WORKED: Biceps (bicep brachii)

12. TRICEP EXTENSION

EASIER VERSION: Stand on the band and grasp both handles together behind your neck. Extend your arms straight overhead while keeping your elbows as close to your ears as possible. Keep your elbows steady and return to the starting position.

HARDER VERSION: Step slightly apart or choose stronger tubing.

MUSCLE WORKED: Triceps (tricep brachii)

Lean Belly Challenge Plan

CIRCUIT	BEGINNER	INTERMEDIATE
# of exercises	6-10	12
# of reps	15	15-20
# of sets (cycles)	1-2	2-3
Rest between exercises	15-60 seconds	0-15 seconds
Rest between cycles	2 minutes	1-2 minutes
Sessions per week	2-3	3
Program length	8-12 weeks	4-6 weeks
Rest between days	48-72 hours	48 hours
Total time	20-30 minutes	30-40 minutes

Stretch at the end of each workout, holding each stretch at least 15 seconds.

Stick with It!

Once you achieve your goal, you need to make sure that you have a maintenance program ready to keep you in shape and in good health.

Make exercise and healthy eating part of your life.

CHAPTER 8

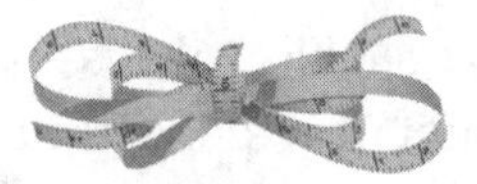

SafSlim™—Nature's Belly Fat Solution

One of the issues with belly fat is how to spot reduce or target fat loss just in the belly region? Up until now, it has been difficult to find the right combination of activity, supplements, and diet to effectively banish that stubborn belly fat. For years, we have known that healthy fats are essential for everything in the body from producing hair, skin, nails, and hormones to reducing inflammation and improving the way our body deals with almost everything. One of the secrets I want to reveal is the belly fat reducing ability of a very common oil—safflower oil.

The seeds that make up safflower oil yield nature's richest source of polyunsaturated fats, including omega-6 and linoleic acid. Today, interest in the health benefits of polyunsaturated oils to lower cholesterol and possibly impact weight control has brought new popularity to this interesting plant. The latest study has shown that safflower oil may have remarkable benefits for belly fat.

A CLOSER LOOK AT SAFFLOWER OIL

Amongst the vegetable oils, safflower oil contains the highest amount of polyunsaturated fats (it is nearly 79% linoleic acid). It also contains about 13% of monounsaturated fatty acids (oleic acid) and 8% saturated fatty acids. Other nutrients found in safflower oil include omega-6 fatty acids, cis-linoleic acid, vitamin E. and phytosterols. The presence of these nutrients and their ratios is likely responsible for the belly fat loss results experienced in the Ohio State study.

Table 1: Polyunsaturated Fatty Acid Composition of Various Oils

NAME OF OIL	% POLYUNSATURATED FAT (linoleic acid)
Safflower	78
Soybean	51
Peanut	32
Canola	21
Olive	10
Palm	2
Coconut	2

Fat to Beat Fat

The idea that fat plays a role in fat loss is difficult to grasp. After all, most of us are under the impression that increasing fat in the diet increases the risk of becoming overweight or obese. However, research is beginning to show that specific types of fat are actually beneficial in helping us lose weight through a number of interesting mechanisms.

High Linoleic Acid Safflower Oil Beats Belly Fat

To have a greater appreciation for safflower oil and to gain a greater understanding of the possible fat-loss mechanisms, a thorough review of a new study published by the *American Journal of Clinical Nutrition (AJCN)* in 2009 is useful. I don't want you to think that it's just me talking about this research because I am not alone; every media outlet seemed to focus on this profound discovery. *Women's World* broke the news in January 2010, which sent a flurry of women into stores looking for safflower oil. Little did they know the kind of oil used in the study was almost virtually impossible to find.

The *AJCN* study involved 35 women who were considered obese based on their BMI values. These women were also postmenopausal and had type 2 diabetes. None of the women took insulin shots for the diabetes; however, many did take medications, such as cholesterol-, blood pressure-, and sugar-managing prescriptions.

Although we've only mentioned safflower oil, the study

actually compared two oils: high linoleic acid safflower oil (unlike the high oleic acid cooking variety) and conjugated linoleic acid (CLA, known to reduce overall body fat).

The women in the study took one of the oils for 16 weeks followed by the other oil for an equal amount of time. In order to ensure that the study was measuring only the effects of the oil supplementation, the participants were instructed not to change their diets or exercise routines over the course of the study.

Among the surprising findings was the fact that about 2 teaspoons of oils rich in linoleic acid had a significant effect on the women's body composition. Women lost between 2 to 4 pounds of belly fat by simply taking high linoleic safflower oil; this translates to about a 6.3% loss. Safflower oil also increased lean tissue (muscle) by an average of about 1.4 pounds and 3 pounds. Translated, this means that women taking safflower oil not only lost belly fat but also gained lean muscle mass (a good thing).

The study also found that the women taking the safflower oil supplements also had lowered fasting blood sugar levels. The participants fasting blood sugar levels dropped between 11 to 19 points (mg/dL) on average, which is considered very significant for type 2 diabetics.

As we've previously mentioned, adiponectin is a protein hormone that modulates a number of metabolic processes, including sugar regulation and the break down of fats (fatty acid catabolism). People with diabetes and obese individuals seem to have lower levels of adiponectin. This study found that women who took safflower oil during the study had increases in adiponectin levels, which may explain how they lost the belly fat.

Although this study opens up great opportunities for people who want to lose belly fat, it also poses a number of important questions. How does safflower actually reduce belly fat? Is this an isolated study, or is there other evidence that helps support these findings and can give us more confidence in this uniquely positioned oil?

Safflower and Weight Loss

Based on current evidence, it would be safe to assume that safflower oil seems to enhance body metabolism, thereby preventing the accumulation of fat in the body. This was supported in the Ohio State study, since safflower oil decreased belly fat and increased lean muscle mass. Both of these observations point toward an increase in metabolism.

The promotion of adiponectin levels (up to a 20% increase) by safflower oil is another important aspect in fat loss. It is well established that adiponectin is a hormone associated with sugar regulation and the breakdown of fat. Research has shown that lower levels of this hormone are found in obese individuals and that increasing circulating levels will have beneficial effects on both weight loss and sugar regulation. Dr. Belury, one of the lead researchers for this study, said that the increased adiponectin levels might have triggered the body's ability to burn dietary fats.

Something important to note is the fact that these

observations were made when people consumed safflower oil irrespective of any changes in their regular diet and exercise program.

Possible Mechanisms of Action

So how is it possible that safflower oil was able to spot reduce belly fat when up until now, it has been difficult to find any natural substance that can target just belly fat? The fact that safflower oil can reduce belly fat, lower fasting sugar levels, and increase lean body mass is pleasantly surprising. "I never would have imagined such a finding. This study is the first to show that such a modest amount of a linoleic-acid-rich oil may have a profound effect on body composition in women," Dr. Belury stated.

There are a number of theories about the health benefits of safflower oil. Reviewing current studies and other ongoing research can help us shed some light into its ability to aid in weight loss and sugar regulation.

Cell Membrane Fluidity

We already discussed the importance of cell membrane fluidity in Chapter 3, but it's worth touching on the subject briefly again to understand safflower oil's fat-reducing ability.

The study of disease processes confirms that changes in cell membrane function are the key factors in the development of virtually every disease. For example, in the Ohio State study, all subjects were type 2 diabetics who also were overweight and carried belly fat. Thus, the improvement in these parameters noted after the safflower supplementation could have been a function of cell membrane fluidity improvements.

When cell membranes become stiff because of the consumption of unhealthy fats, cells lose their ability to hold nutrients, electrolytes, and even water. The lack of fluidity in the membranes also impairs their ability to communicate with other cells and affects how they are influenced by hormones, such as insulin. For example, hormones and communicating molecules that increase the ability of the cells to burn energy or fat may be impeded; the end result is a slowdown of metabolism and an accumulation of fat within the cell.

Although the exact mechanism of action is still unknown, increasing cell membrane fluidity with safflower oil could be one of the mechanisms by which blood sugar is lowered. The increase in fluidity allows more movement of insulin receptor sites on cell membranes and, therefore, an improvement in the ability of insulin to bind to them. This increase in affinity is a possible contributing factor to the effects of safflower oil.

As noted, improving cell membrane fluidity can bring cell membranes back to healthy functionality. This can be done by changes in dietary habits and supplementing with healthy fats, such as safflower oil. Patience is important because it takes months for these polyunsaturated fats to become incorporated in cells and have positive effects.

Note that in the Ohio State study, it was a 16-week time frame that resulted in positive changes.

Brown Fat Connection

Brown fat is present in several areas of the body, and its main function is to produce heat, known as thermogenesis. This action is the major factor making brown fat activation favorable for weight loss. It seems that cis-linoleic acid, a fatty acid present in safflower oils, gets converted into gamma linolenic acid (GLA), which in turn triggers brown fat to burn calories. Originally, studies into this area were carried out by Dr. David Horrobin of the University of Montreal. Using GLA, he found that subjects with metabolic weight loss problems could be helped by giving this oil in supplement form. The observations were that GLA stimulated brown fat to start burning fat. This may be another way that safflower oil contributes to belly fat loss and lean body muscle gain.

Enhanced Blood Sugar Control

Linoleic acid enhances blood sugar control by increasing insulin-producing cells' sensitivity to sugar. As this study demonstrated, a drop in the fasting blood sugar levels of subjects who took safflower oil was significant and could be useful for the enormous pre-diabetic population in the United States (pre-diabetes occurs when a person's fasting blood sugar falls between 100 mg/dL and 125 mg/dL). To give you some perspective, there are about 57 million pre-diabetics in the United States with another 23 million having already being diagnosed with diabetes. That means that there are over 80 million Americans who have sugar-regulating problems. Most of these individuals could benefit from polyunsaturated fatty acid supplementation.

Some interesting new research being done in the biotechnology sector may shed more light onto the possible mechanisms of action of this plant. The pharmaceutical company SemiBiosys Genetics is currently using a type of safflower oil to produce human insulin. Human insulin derived from Safflower oil is currently going through Phase I and II trials on human test subjects. Currently, Humulin® is being used to treat Type I diabetics. Developing an efficiently low-cost substitute from safflower oil could significantly change treatment options for people all over the world not able to afford modern insulin costs.

What's interesting is that within the safflower family of molecules, there are structures similar to human insulin. Could this be one of the ways by which safflower oil has the ability to lower fasting blood sugar levels? Although nothing has been confirmed, this could be another plausible mechanism of action.

Adiponectin

As already discussed, one of the findings from the current research on safflower oil is its ability to increase adiponectin levels. Research has shown that overweight and obese individuals have lower levels of adiponectin as do type 2 diabetics. Adiponectin released from fat cells is a hormone that improves insulin sensitivity and can help mobilize belly fat. The goal is to have high levels of adiponectin, so the less fat you have, the more adiponectin is released. If you have a lot of belly fat, there will be only a small amount of adiponectin released, which causes your cells to become resistant to insulin and, in turn, will cause more fat to be stored in the belly region. Adiponectin also has anti-inflammatory effects on the cells lining the walls of the blood vessels. High blood levels of adiponectin are associated with a reduced risk of heart attack.

Current research has shown that consuming safflower daily over a 16-week period can increase adiponectin levels by 20%. This is significant because of the actions adiponectin has on body metabolism and weight loss. For one, adiponectin may impact the expression of various genes that can turn on cells to begin the breakdown of fats. This is possibly linked to a complex network of reactions involving PPAR-alpha (peroxisome proliferator activator receptors). One possible result of all this is the increase in mitochondria found in skeletal muscles. Mitochondria are energy-producing factories; the more mitochondria within cells, the more energy being produced. Because Adiponectin may increasre the amount of mitochondria in muscle cells, it is likely that it enhances energy production in the body and directly affects metabolism.

This is a very powerful effect associated with safflower oil supplementation, and could be the main thrust of this supplement's effects on belly fat.

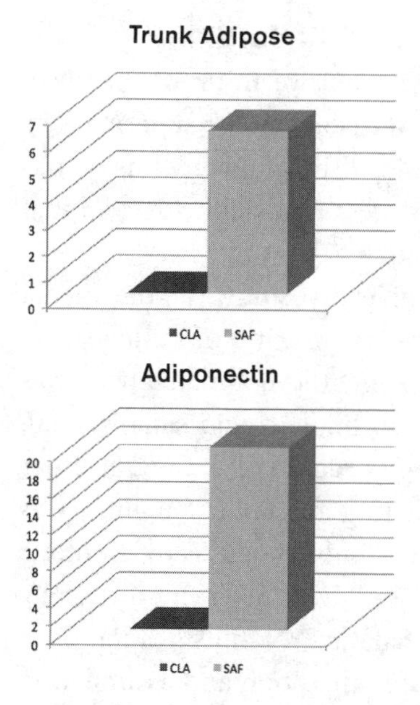

Linoleic Acid Helps to Decrease Inflammation

The omega-6 fatty acid linoleic acid gets converted into gamma linolenic acid (GLA), which further metabolizes into our body's very important anti-inflammatory hormones. In fact, GLA has been shown to be one of nature's most valuable anti-inflammatory agents. In fact, it is so potent that it has proven to be useful for many conditions, including eczema, psoriasis, and rheumatoid arthritis.

Systemic inflammation has been shown to promote fat storage. Most North Americans are living with a constant state of inflammation raging through their bodies. Inflammation begins with a poor diet high in processed foods, trans fats, sugar, and alcohol. This causes excess insulin, which fuels the inflammatory process in the body.

Safflower oil has been shown to decrease inflammation in the body, which in turn could be a possible mechanism for the mobilization of stored fat. The less inflammation, the less fat storage.

High Linoleic Acid Safflower Oil SafSlim™

When we think of safflower oil, we think of the clear, flavorless oil commercially available in all supermarkets for a relatively inexpensive price. Unfortunately this oil has been highly refined, which creates an unstable toxic oil that is unhealthy for us to consume.

When the Ohio State University study hit the media world, women ran to find the "right" kind of safflower oil, but of course, what they could find did not match what was studied. The study used a high linoleic acid safflower oil, which is not readily available. In order to meet the consumer demand created by this exciting research, SafSlim™ was developed. To make safflower oil more body ready, a unique patented form of emulsified safflower oil is commercially available under the name SafSlim™. Emulsification is a technology that allows for rapid digestion and assimilation through the intestinal tract and into the bloodstream, thus allowing for maximum cellular bioavailability that is far superior to the oil in its natural form. Considering the state of most North American's gastrointestinal and digestive systems, there are so many variables that can prevent the proper assimilation of oils; therefore, oil available in a pre-emulsified form will help improve bioavailability.

By supplementing with safflower oil, establishing a healthy nutrition plan and food choices, and implanting the exercises recommended in this book, we can all be successful at banishing belly fat.

Belly Fat Breakthrough

— RESOURCES —

Belly Fat Breakthrough Website

For additional information, recipes, newsletter, detailed fitness exercises, and support, go to

www.bellyfatbreakthroughbook.com

Follow us on Twitter

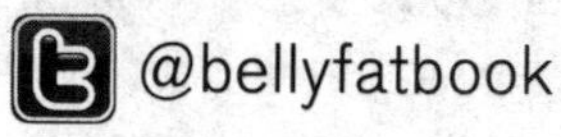

Lose Belly Fat with Nature's True Belly Fat Solution!

For more information, go to

www.safslim.com

KARLENE KARST, RD

Karlene Karst, RD, is a leading health specialist in nutrition and natural medicine. She is the coauthor of the national bestseller *Healthy Fats for Life* and author of *The Metabolic Syndrome Program*. These are all part of Karlene's efforts to encourage people to get "back to the basics" of nutrition. Karlene holds a BS in Nutrition from the University of Saskatchewan in Canada and is a registered dietitian. Karlene is a highly sought-after, enthusiastic, and passionate individual and is a frequent guest speaker at educational events and on radio and TV shows around North America. www.karlenekarst.com.

INGRID VADINA

Ingrid Vadina grew up in Slovakia and has been living in Vancouver, British Columbia, since 1996. She has always had a passion for fitness and became a BCRPA Certified Personal Trainer. Ingrid is also an indoor cycling instructor and fitness competitor. She worked for Steve Nash Fitness World from 2001 to 2010, but in early 2011, she decided to start her own personal training business, Fit & Strong.

As a mother of two, Ingrid understands that staying healthy and fit is necessary to have energy for balancing a busy life. "I have truly found what I love to do for living," Ingrid revealed "and now is my opportunity to help others improve their health and quality of life through exercise. I love helping my clients reach their goals!"